Healthy Eating

3rd Edition

55 POWERFUL Eating Habits That Will Keep You Healthy & Feeling Energized!

by Linda Westwood

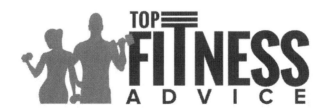

Linda Westwood
TopFitnessAdvice.com

Table of Contents

Who is this book for?

Do you feel like the food you eat just makes you tired and lazy every day?

Are you struggling to stick to healthy habits and lose weight?

Are you one of those people who *know* what to do, but struggle to *actually do* it?

Then this book is for you!

I am going to share with you some of the MOST effective eating habits that you can add into your life to lose weight, feel great and have LOTS of energy!

I have given you a simple action plan at the end of each Healthy Eating Habit so you can implement each habit very easily!

Also, you don't have to be overweight to benefit from these habits.

Yes, they help you lose weight, but they also help you live a healthy life, as well as feel energized throughout your day!

What will this book teach you?

This book is not like others!

It doesn't just contain generic advice that we all already know, but actual eating habits that have been identified to INCREASE weight loss, IMPROVE energy levels, and lead to a more HEALTHY life!

Some of these habits are very simple and you can begin implementing them today, and some are a little more difficult, in that you will need to practice them more!

I will also share with you why each of these habits work and are so effective – along with a simple action plan to help get you started and on your way to lasting success!

Healthy Eating Habit 1: Eat Healthy Unprocessed Food

For many of us, time is a commodity that is in short supply. We work harder than ever before, and more often than not, we look for shortcuts wherever we can.

And the stores make it that much easier for us, don't they?

It's simple to pick up a tray of peeled and chopped veggies, or a ready-made meal to either zap in the microwave or to heat through in the oven.

Dinner can be on the table in minutes instead of hours.

It's great, isn't it?

Why Processed Foods Should Be an Occasional Indulgence

Processed foods are convenient, but they are not the healthy solution we think that they are. What you have to remember is that food deteriorates quite quickly after it is prepared, especially if it is exposed to oxygen.

You've probably seen it happen yourself a number of times at home. For example, when you cut an apple it starts to go brown almost immediately.

The same thing happens to prepared foods, but the manufacturer knows that the product must still look good so that you will buy it. They know that you are not going to look kindly on discolored vegetables or food that looks less than perfect.

They also want their product to have the best possible shelf life and taste, and this can be where the real problems come in.

Preservatives, Colorants, Fats and Sugar

Preservatives, colorants, fats, and sugar are the processed food manufacturers go-to products. The preservatives extend the shelf life of the food, the colorants make it look better, and the fats and sugar are used to make it taste better.

Try this experiment for yourself:

Buy organic lettuce from the local farmer's market and buy a salad pack from one of the grocery stores. Put both in the refrigerator and see which lasts longer. The organic one will start to wilt in a few days time. This is normal. The salad pack, on the other hand, will probably still look great after a week, sometimes even two weeks.

Many pre-prepared cut vegetables and fruit are soaked in chlorinated water to prevent them from decaying as quickly. Those perfectly shaped little baby carrots that you buy pre-peeled are actually normal carrots that have been pushed through a cutter to make them look "mini."

Not only are you taking in a lot more chemicals with the pre-prepared options, but you also have no real idea how nutritious the food is. The longer it sits on the shelf, the worse it is nutritionally.

Now, we are going to talk a little about the fats and sugars added to processed foods. Processing food removes a lot of nutrients and flavor. Take a pot of beans on the stove, for example. The longer they are cooked, the mushier and less appetizing they become. The same principle applies to processed foods.

The manufacturers know that the key to making the food taste good lies in adding fat and sugar. And let's face it, they are right. Fat and sugar do taste good.

The problem with this is that we usually have no idea how much extra fat and sugar we are getting when we eat packaged foods. After all, how many of us read the labels?

And how many of us actually realize that reduced fat foods are the worst culprits? Just take a look at the label of any low-fat yogurt, for example. I'll bet that sugar is in the top 3 listed ingredients.

What You Can Do

The truth is that it that you should really only eat processed foods every now and again, if at all. Avoiding them is not as hard as you may think. It's just a matter of breaking the habit of relying on them.

You just need to start prepping your own food and looking for creative ways to minimize preparation time. Cook double quantities and freeze half. Find the freshest veggies and fruit, and eat them raw.

Consider the peeled and cubed butternut squash that you just pop in the pot and boil. You can simply buy a whole butternut squash. Peeling it takes a few minutes, but if you are not up for that, just cut it in half, scoop out the seeds, and roast it in the oven.

What you really want to do is start eating food as close to its natural state as possible. Experiment with new ways to prepare food in smart ways to cut down on the prep work. The fresher the food, the better the flavor, so the less seasoning you need to add. Your food will taste better and be a lot healthier with a little bit of extra effort.

By preparing your own meals, you can control exactly what goes into them.

Action Plan

- Find a local farmer's market and select fresh produce. This goes for eggs, milk, bread, veggies, etc.

- Get yourself a packet of Ziploc freezer bags.

- Get yourself a permanent marker.

- Read up on cooking for the freezer.

- Whenever you make your favorite dish, double the quantity and freeze half for later use.

- Consider setting some time at the weekend aside for preparing and cooking meals that can be frozen. Voila! You now have your own convenience foods at a fraction of the cost.

Healthy Eating Habit 2: Switch to Healthy Whole Grains

According to a study conducted by the University of Copenhagen in 2012, when overweight people ate more whole grains, they lost more weight than those who did not eat the whole grains. They also improved their cholesterol levels.

The sad truth today is that very few of us get enough fiber on a daily basis. The Western diet is notorious for being high in refined carbohydrates and low in fiber.

The problem with refined carbohydrates is that they are so easy for the body to convert to glucose in the blood stream. As a result, after eating, the bloodstream is flooded with glucose, and you experience an energy spike. The body goes into emergency mode to mop this up with insulin, and so your energy crashes. The end result is that you feel hungry again in a couple of hours.

If this occurs once in a while, it's not a problem. If it occurs on a regular basis, the body's insulin response becomes damaged and less effective. You start to develop insulin resistance, and eventually, Type II diabetes.

What You Can Do

Fortunately, the solution is fairly simple. You need to add more wholegrain foods to your diet.

This can be as simple as buying brown rice instead of white or choosing whole wheat pasta over the refined version.

Start incorporating more low GI grains into your diet, and avoid highly refined foods so that your energy levels remain consistent.

Action Plan

- Go to your local library or bookstore, or run an online search for more information about the Glycemic Index.

- Make a list of foods, including whole grains, which you can incorporate into your diet and that fit into the lower half of the Glycemic Index.

- Always choose the less refined version of any product that you are considering buying.

Read This FIRST - 100% FREE BONUS

FOR A LIMITED TIME ONLY – Get Linda's best-selling book *"Quick & Easy Weight Loss: 97 Scientifically Proven Tips Even For Those With Busy Schedules!"* absolutely FREE!

Readers who have read this bonus book along with this book have seen the greatest changes in their weight loss both *FAST & EASILY* and have improved overall fitness levels – so it is *highly recommended* to get this bonus book.

Once again, as a big thank-you for downloading this book, I'd like to offer it to you *100% FREE for a LIMITED TIME ONLY!*

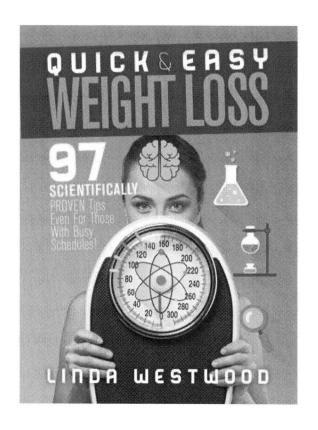

Get your free copy at:

TopFitnessAdvice.com/Bonus

Healthy Eating Habit 3: Start Cooking in Healthy Ways

My grandma taught me a bit about cooking, and to this day, those lessons have stuck with me. I always cook pork chops in the oven for at least an hour in case the meat is contaminated.

Now, this was a problem in my grandma's day, but really isn't anymore. Still, the lessons she taught persist. I boil veggies until they are soft, and I always add sugar and butter when cooking carrots.

I am sure that you have learned some bad habits when it comes to cooking as well.

Maybe you also boil veggies until they are mushy and colorless. Is it any wonder why you're not excited to eat them?

What You Can Do

You need to start looking into healthier ways to prepare food and to avoid extremely unhealthy ones such as deep fat frying.

Make as much of your own food as possible so that you know exactly what is in it.

Healthy Cooking Can Taste Good

There is also a perception out there that healthy cooking methods can produce tasteless foods. If you're willing to do a little research, you'll find that the opposite is actually true.

Start off with fresh, high-quality ingredients. You have just won the first half of the battle to make your food taste great.

Many vegetables can either be eaten raw or lightly steamed. There is really no reason to boil them. In fact, if they retain their crunch, they add an interesting texture to the meal. Sprinkle with a bit of butter or some lemon juice to really up the taste factor.

It is also a good idea to experiment with different herbs and spices so that you can reduce your reliance on salt. Growing your own herbs is easy and can be a great incentive for you to use them while cooking.

Stir-frying meat and vegetables in a small amount of olive oil is a simple and effective way to get tasty and healthy meals.

Also, consider grilling your food. Grilled food often ends up tasting more flavorful, and the process is more natural.

No More Deep Fat Frying

There is no place in the healthy kitchen for deep fat frying.

The high heat temperatures cause chemical changes in the oils that make them dangerous trans-fatty acids.

These trans-fats contribute significantly to inflammation and disease.

Make Your Own Sauces

This is possibly the best tip in this section. It is not that difficult to make a simple vinaigrette or tomato-based sauce, and it is a great way to add tons of flavor without all the additives found in store-bought sauces.

Action Plan

- Look over your favorite family recipes and see how they can be made healthier. What about grilling that steak instead of frying it, or baking the chicken instead of deep-frying it?

- Research recipes that involve steaming or stir-frying your food.

- Whenever possible, eat your food raw. Perhaps have carrot crudités instead of boiled carrots.

- Start experimenting with different spices when it comes to preparing your food.

- Find ways to make your own sauces to use on salads, pastas, etc.

Healthy Eating Habit 4: Always Eat Healthy Portions

It is a well-known fact that portion sizes have truly gotten out of hand. You are actively encouraged to supersize your meal in order to get the best possible deal, and portion sizes at restaurants seem to keep getting bigger and bigger.

Most of us are eating far too much food, even if we only have one helping. We tend to be confused about what the right portion sizes are. After all, when you go to a restaurant, you think that they know what they are doing, right?

They do know what they are doing. They are making you think that you are getting the best value at their restaurant. The bigger portion size is more about good business sense than any desire to serve healthy food.

But restaurants teach this behavior, and you take it into your daily life. So, you dish out much larger portions that you should.

What You Can Do

Fortunately, getting back to properly sized portions is pretty easy. Start by taking your dinner plate and dividing it into four quarters.

One quarter of the plate should contain your protein. The next quarter should be your low GI starches or carbohydrates, and the rest of the plate should be filled with low-carb vegetables.

Ideally speaking, lunch or breakfast should be the main meal of the day, and dinner should be the smallest meal.

Action Plan

- Start by tracing one of your dinner plates onto a piece of paper.

- Divide this drawing up into four equal quarters.

- Take measurements if needed so that you know exactly how much food you can add per quarter.

- Look for smaller plates from which to eat your dinner.

- Consult your GI list to find carbohydrates with a score of 50 or less to use as a starch.

Healthy Eating Habit 5: Healthy Ways to Eat Out

Many dieters try to avoid eating out whenever possible. It's simply too tempting to eat in a restaurant.

It is harder to make healthier choices when eating out, especially when you are with a bunch of friends who are encouraging you to join in and skip the diet.

The portion sizes in a restaurant can also be a problem.

At the same time, you don't want to sit at home night after night and miss out on the fun with your friends.

What you Can Do

Fortunately, it is not an insurmountable problem.

Keeping the portioning advice in mind, start by looking online to see what the restaurant has on the menu that's relatively healthy. Pay particular attention to the entrees.

Nothing is stopping you from ordering an entrée with a side salad as your main meal. With the salad, order the dressing on the side and add a little, not a lot.

If that is not an option, always choose vegetables or rice as an alternative to chips, and ask the waiter to box up half of your meal to go immediately. This can be taken home for another day.

And always remember that you do not have to finish all the food on your plate. You are an adult now; you can decide exactly how much, or how little, you want to eat.

Action Plan

- Start researching restaurants in your area and see how flexible they are willing to be. When your friends want to go out, suggest restaurants that are more suitable for your diet based on your research.

- Ask the waiter how dishes are prepared, and ask for sauces and salad dressings to be served on the side.

- If items are cooked in butter, you can request that they are cooked in olive oil instead.

- Most restaurants will allow you to switch out you chips for a salad, so you should ask if this is possible.

- Be prepared for a little ribbing from your friends, but also be prepared to stand your ground. If they don't worry about their health, that's their choice. But they don't have any right to make you feel bad about taking care of yours.

Healthy Eating Habit 6: Start Using a Food Diary

How much have you eaten today? What about yesterday? I bet you think you can list it accurately.

Did you include the sugar from the cup of coffee you drank or the spoonful of soup you tasted while making supper?

Research has shown that we tend to underestimate the amount of food that we eat on any given day.

This can lead to problems when it comes to understanding weight gain. You might genuinely believe that you have followed a healthy eating plan all week and be at a loss as to why you have gained, rather than lost, weight.

What You Can Do

The simple answer is to keep a food diary. This may seem like a bit of a pain at first, but there are a number of reasons why it is helpful.

- You record everything that you eat so you have an accurate record of caloric intake.

- You are more aware of the amounts that you are eating and are more focused on what you are eating. You might be less inclined to sample the cheese when you're grating it if you know you'll have to write it in your diary.

- You can identify trigger situations and eating patterns and learn how to work around them.

Action Plan

- Buy a small notebook today. It should be something that can be easily carried in your purse or pocket. Also, keep a little pen to go with it.

- As soon as you eat anything, make a note. There is no point of leaving it until later, since you might forget.

- Also, record how you were feeling when you ate.
- If you want to, you can total up the calories at the end of the day. This might be useful, but it is not necessary.

- Look for patterns that emerge. Maybe you always eat chips when watching your favorite TV show, for example.

Healthy Eating Habit 7: Plan Your Shopping in Advance

It is too easy to just order takeout when you are not in the mood to cook.

At other times, you want to make something healthy but don't have the ingredients. So, you go shopping while you are hungry or rushing. This is a huge mistake, and can lead to purchases you'll regret.

What You Can Do

Set aside time once a week to make a complete shopping list and then set aside a time to go shopping. Make sure that you are not hungry when you go shopping, and do not deviate from the list.

Include healthy foods that can easily be turned into a meal. This way, when you are not in the mood for cooking, getting the ingredients and putting them on the stove is actually as easy as ordering takeout.

Action Plan

- Make a standard, weekly grocery list and keep a copy on your computer. That way, all you need to do is add in any extras that you might need for the week, print the list, and go. This will make planning a breeze.

26

- Incorporate ingredients for "lazy" meals (meals that do not require a lot of preparation), for those days when you cannot face cooking.

- Keep a notepad on or near the fridge so that your family can make a note of items that are finished and need replacing.

- Never shop on an empty stomach. Plan your shopping trip when you are relaxed and unhurried.

Healthy Eating Habit 8: Still Eat Treats

As every dieter knows, nothing is more desirable than a food that you are not allowed to eat.

If you have been having sweets and other favorite foods on a regular basis and then suddenly have to give them up completely, there is a better than average chance that you are going to crave them and will eventually give in.

What You Can Do

In order to prevent you from falling off the wagon completely, you should incorporate some of your favorite foods into your eating plan in moderation.

Knowing that you can have a bit of ice cream or some chips once a week will help you stick to your diet because you won't feel as restricted.

Action Plan

- List your favorite foods. They are the foods that you don't think that you could go without forever.

- These foods are not completely banned, but you shouldn't keep them readily available in the house, either.

- Set up a regular day where you are allowed to eat a bit of what you really enjoy.

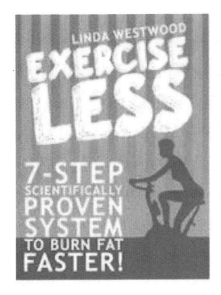
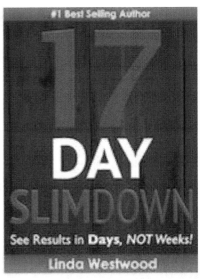
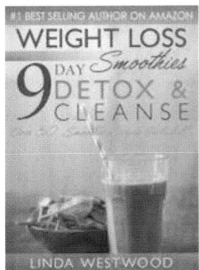
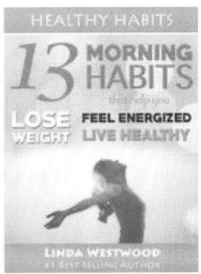

Check out Linda's books at:

TopFitnessAdvice.com/go/books

Healthy Eating Habit 9: Water, Nothing Beats It!

Water is the lifeblood of this planet. Without it, nothing would be able to survive here. Water is incredibly important to us as well. That is why our bodies are made up of 70% water.

Water is an integral part of all the body's processes and you have to make sure that you drink enough of it every single day.

Most of us drink far too little water daily. Consequently, we go through life mildly dehydrated.

What You Can Do

It's not that hard to get enough water. All you need is around two liters a day.

The best way to ensure that you get enough is to get yourself a water bottle, and make a point of emptying it until you are drinking enough every day.

You can add fruits or herbs to it for a bit of extra flavor if you like. Just don't add sugar.

Action Plan

- Buy yourself a water bottle today; glass or aluminum is best.

- Work out how many times you will need to empty the bottle in order to get your full two liters of water each day.

- If desired, flavor it with chopped fruits or herbs.

- Other drinks you have throughout the day, like tea and coffee, do not count toward your total.

Healthy Eating Habit 10: Always Eat Breakfast

Breakfast is the most important meal of the day.

Research has proven repeatedly that people who skip breakfast more than make up for that fact by eating a lot more calories throughout the rest of the day.

Your metabolism needs a jumpstart in the morning, and breakfast is the best way to provide this.

What You Can Do

Follow the same principles for a healthy breakfast as you would for a healthy lunch or dinner. You need some protein, some low GI starches, and fruits and vegetables.

The protein and the fiber in the starch will help you to feel fuller for longer and give you the boost of energy needed to get through your busy morning.

Choose simple, easy to prepare breakfasts. Get up a little earlier if you need to, but always make breakfast a priority.

An example of a good breakfast could be a bowl of oatmeal (starch), a small tub of yogurt (protein), and an apple (fruit).

You don't need a huge breakfast, just a well-balanced one.

Action Plan

- Research some simple and easy to prepare breakfasts.

- Do as much of the prep the night before as you can manage.

- Have at least one quick, eat-on-the-run breakfast plan for those days when you are really running late (a handful of nuts, a piece of fruit, and some oat bars, for example).

Healthy Eating Habit 11: Hit Your Fruit & Vegetable Requirements

You probably know that we are supposed to eat 5 portions of fruits and vegetables a day.

What you might not know, however, is that researchers now believe that that figure should be closer to 9 portions daily for optimal health.

Most people get one or two portions a day, at best.

The problem with this is that it means that most people are missing essential nutrients and fiber. These are things that simply cannot be replaced by taking a vitamin supplement.

We cannot copy the nutrients present in fruits and veggies, but that that is only half of the overall story. Vitamins and minerals in natural sources are hardly ever found in isolation and it is believed that the actual specific interplay of these nutrients within nature is crucial to the body's absorption of all of the nutrients it needs.

We cannot, at this stage, replicate this complex interplay of nutrients. So, it is best to get as many of them naturally as possible.

What You Can Do

Five to nine servings may sound like a lot but it is actually not as bad as it sounds. A medium-sized apple or one cup of cauliflower counts as a single serving.

On the bright side, fruits and vegetables are usually lower on the GI scale and have enough fiber to help keep you feeling fuller for longer.

If you do not make any other changes to your diet, make sure that you get 5-9 portions of fruits and vegetables every day. You will find that you feel fuller and have less of an appetite for junk food. Your caloric intake will decrease naturally.

Action Plan

- Make a list of your favorite fruits and vegetables, and learn what constitutes a portion of each.

- Put them on your standard weekly shopping list. The fresher they are, the better they taste.

- Experiment with different ways to prepare them so that you can incorporate them into your daily diet.

Healthy Eating Habit 12: Sit Down at the Table to Eat

When was the last time you sat down at the table to eat? (A TV tray table doesn't count!)

Many people have developed the extremely bad habit of sitting down to eat on the couch in front of the TV, or eating on the run. Maybe you don't want to miss your favorite show or you are running late for work.

Your mother was right. You should eat at the table.

First of all, eating at table allows you to adopt a better posture when it comes to eating. Secondly, it allows you to be more mindful of what you eat.

How many times have you been eating a bag of popcorn in front of the TV and "suddenly" found that it was finished? The problem with eating in front of the TV is that we can eat a great deal more without even realizing it.

What You Can Do

Eating at the table slows things down and allows for less distraction. It is also a good way for a family to reconnect with one another on a daily basis.

Action Plan

- Clear off the dining room table, and pull out your placemats.

- Get everyone into the habit of eating meals at the table.

- It can be a nice ritual to dress the table for special occasions.

Healthy Eating Habit 13: Always Carry a Protein-Rich Snack

No matter how healthy your diet is, there is always a chance that you might start to feel a little hungry between meals. The problem with ignoring that slight hunger is that it grows until you feel as though you are starving.

And then, you just about inhale your food and eat a lot more than you actually should.

What You Can Do

Carrying around a protein-rich snack makes good sense. Protein is one of the most satiating foods. Even eating one egg can help to tide you over until your next meal.

Protein also gives you a much-needed energy boost.

Pre-empting the hunger pangs by having a protein-rich snack can go a long way toward helping you follow a healthy eating plan.

Action Plan

- List all the protein sources that you can think of that would serve as good and practical snacks. You could, for example, keep a tin of tuna or a packet of nuts in your desk drawer.

- Plan to incorporate snack times into your day. Now that you have analyzed your food diary, you should know when optimal snacking times are throughout the day.

- Plan your snacks at regular intervals. You should not go more than 3-4 hours without eating.

Healthy Eating Habit 14: Have A Green Tea After Meals

Unfortunately, the world is full of toxins. There are toxins in the food we eat, the water we drink, and even air that we breathe.

Add in the fact that few of us get enough fruits and vegetables (thus, we miss out on the anti-oxidants that they provide), and it comes as no surprise that we are battling oxidative stress, which contributes to premature aging and serious illness.

What You Can Do

You can help boost your anti-oxidant levels and energy levels safely and naturally by having a cup of green tea after every meal. Green tea (without milk) is an excellent source of anti-oxidants.

It also contains a healthy dose of caffeine, less than the amount found in coffee, which can help boost energy levels without causing the "jitters."

Action Plan

- Buy a box of green tea today.

- Keep a box at home and a box at the office.

- If the weather is hot, you can make a refreshing green iced tea and keep it in the refrigerator.

Healthy Eating Habit 15: Always Carry a Water Bottle

As mentioned above, we need to drink 2 liters of water a day. Most people don't get nearly enough.

What You Can Do

Always having water on hand will make it that much easier to remember to drink your 2 liters a day. Keep the bottle on your desk and sip whenever you remember to.

Action Plan

- Get yourself a bottle for water and make sure to place it where you can see it throughout the day.

- Promise yourself at the start of each day that you will drink sufficient water and force yourself to reach your quota. Soon, it will become a habit.

Healthy Eating Habit 16: Combine Carbohydrates & Protein

There was a movement a while back called "food combining." It was theorized that different enzymes were needed to digest carbohydrates and proteins.

Research has since proven that this is complete nonsense, but there are some people that adhere to the basic principles.

The problem with eating just one or the other is that you are basically not getting enough food to feel satisfied.

Let's say, for example, you have a few slices of toast for breakfast without any protein to slow down the release of glucose into the bloodstream, you are going to feel hungry again in a couple of hours.

Conversely, if you just eat an egg for breakfast, there really isn't enough food to help you to feel full.

What You Can Do

Carbohydrates provide fiber and protein helps you feel fuller. They are the perfect meal combination.

Action Plan

- Plan your meals around the principles laid out above. Plan to always eat a carbohydrate (starch) and protein at each meal and snack.

- Research some easy combinations that you can turn to in a pinch. For example, an apple and a handful of almonds make an energizing and filling snack.

Healthy Eating Habit 17: Try to Eat Small & Nutritious Meals Often

Many of us snack throughout the day. We are natural grazers. The problem is that the snacks we choose are often not very healthy.

Most of us, at some time or another, have raided the office vending machine for a high calorie snack, only to feel even hungrier a few hours later.

What You Can Do

"Grazing," (having smaller, more frequent meals), is a good idea. The key is to have high-quality meals and snacks. You should not go longer than 3-4 hours without a meal or a snack.

If you do not allow yourself to get hungry, you are always able to control your food choices. If you get very hungry, you are likely to binge eat, or turn to something unhealthy.

Choosing nutritious food makes sense. You want your body to have the very best fuel, don't you?

Action Plan

- Always buy the best quality foods that you can get. The better the quality and the fresher the food, the better the flavor is.

- The body does better with a steady flow of energy. Plan your day properly with breakfast, lunch, supper, and a snack in between each of these.

Healthy Eating Habit 18: Never Let Yourself Become Too Hungry

Many dieters mistakenly believe that skipping meals will help them to lose weight. It seems to make sense. If you only eat two meals a day, you eat less calories overall.

The problem is that your body catches on to what you are doing quite quickly and becomes sneaky. It will make you eat more in order to make up for the calories loss.

Worse still, the hungrier you are, the less control you have over what you eat. Your body will crave the high calorie foods because it is going into defense mode.

You will not only be more likely to binge, but more likely to binge on high calorie junk food.

What You Can Do

The key is to never activate the body's defenses against starvation. In order to do this, you need to ensure that you eat enough so that you don't ever feel starving.

This means planning your day, as well as your meals and snacks, carefully.

Action Plan

- Always start the day with a good, balanced breakfast.

- Pack a balanced lunch and snacks, as well.

- Have an emergency snack supply for use should the need arise.

- Make sure that you make healthy choices that help you to feel fuller longer.

Healthy Eating Habit 19: Eat Slowly & Chew Thoroughly

How often do you gulp down your food as fast as you can?

Most of us eat far too fast and don't even bother to chew our food properly. There was once a piece of advice doing the rounds that it was necessary to chew your food at least a hundred times over.

What You Can Do

Now, chewing 100 times is taking it too far. But the principle is that you should chew your food properly. It takes about 20 minutes for the brain to actually recognize that you have eaten enough.

Eating slowly gives your brain and body time to catch up. You will end up eating less overall.

Chewing your food properly makes the digestive process smoother for two reasons. First, the stomach is more easily able to break the food down. Second, less air is swallowed during the meal, reducing excess gas.

Action Plan

- Make eating a ritual rather than a hurried affair.

- Sit down to eat at a table, and never hurry through your meal mindlessly.

- Take the time to chew each bite properly before swallowing.

- Eat with a knife and fork and put these down after each bite to slow down the rate at which you eat.

Healthy Eating Habit 20: Colorful is Better

In nature, different colors point to different properties. In food, the color indicates the presence of different nutrients.

Humans tend to be creatures of habit. We often eat the same foods day in and day out.

Nutritionally, this can mean that we do not get the range of nutrients that we require for optimal health.

What You Can Do

Varying your diet can be exciting and also very healthy for you.

Making sure that you eat a range of fruits and vegetables across the color spectrum increases your chances of getting the right mix of essential nutrients.

Action Plan

- If possible, start growing your own greens so that you have a variety at hand when you need them. Alternatively, find a good, organic source of fruits and vegetables.

- Rethink what part of the plant is edible. Carrot greens, for example, can be extremely nutritious. You have orange and green in one basic veggie.

- Vary the produce that you buy. If you bought apples this week, for example, buy pears next week.

Healthy Eating Habit 21: Cut Down on Sugars

Did you know that the most common ingredient in processed foods is sugar?

I was horrified to find out that sugar is used in the curing of bacon and in the making of smoked chicken as well.

Take a look at the labels of the foods that you eat. Even if you are not adding a single spoonful of sugar to anything that you eat, there is a good chance that you are eating too much of it anyway.

Sugar is non-nutritive and highly addictive. It causes the brain to release endorphins. That is why eating chocolate is such a pleasurable experience.

The overconsumption of sugar has been linked to an increase in Type II Diabetes, obesity, and heart disease.

What You Can Do

What you need to do is to break your addiction to sugar as soon as possible. You need to bring your blood sugar levels back under control.

Fortunately, a lot of the damage done by sugar can be reversed. You do, however, need to acknowledge that sugar is an addiction just like any other. The best way to get over it is to cut it out completely.

Cut out all sugar and added sugar for at least two weeks, and you will break your addiction.

Action Plan

- Check the labels of all the foods that you currently have in your kitchen cabinets. You'll be surprised how much sugar is added.

- Read the labels of any foods that you plan to buy. The higher up on the list of ingredients that sugar is labeled, the higher the sugar content is. Avoid foods with sugar listed in the top 5 ingredients.

- Do not bother with artificial sweeteners. They do not fool the body, and can actually fuel cravings for sugar. A sweet tooth is a taste that is learned. It can be unlearned as well.

Healthy Eating Habit 22: Eat More Fish & Nuts

Fish is one of those foods that you either love or you hate. There does not really seem to be a middle ground here. Those of us who do not like eating fish know that it is good for us but are not often swayed by that logic.

Nuts are a food that many of us enjoy but are very scared to eat because we were raised believing that they were extremely fattening.

The problem is that both fish, especially oily fish, and nuts are rich in essential fatty acids that we simply cannot get anywhere else. They are present in plant sources, but not in a form that our bodies can efficiently use.

These Omega-3 fatty acids are essential in the fight against inflammation and pain.

What You Can Do

Oily fish, like salmon, should be on the menu at least twice a week in order to get a sufficient quantity of Omega-3 fatty acids.

If you really cannot bring yourself to include fish in your diet, you need to take a cod liver oil supplement every day.

Nuts are high in calories but they are also packed with energy, protein, healthy fats, and fiber. Nuts are great to keep on hand as a healthy snack.

The key is to monitor your intake. You only need a handful a day at most.

Action Plan

- Buy a bag of nuts and divide it into individual portion sizes.

- Nuts are a great addition to salads. Chop them up, and sprinkle them on top.

- If you do enjoy fish, research new recipes and ways to prepare it.

- If you do not enjoy fish, find a good quality cod liver oil supplement, and take it daily.

Healthy Eating Habit 23: Limit Animal Fats

Many of us were raised to believe that a balanced meal consisted of meat, a starch, and vegetables. We are definitely a meat-eating nation, and there is nothing wrong with that.

The reality is that we eat far too much meat. A portion of meat should be no bigger or thicker than the palm of your hand but we regularly consume pieces two or three times that size.

The problem is not the meat itself, but the fats the meat contains. Who doesn't enjoy a nice piece of roast pork?

These saturated fats can be very damaging to your health. They have been linked with increased cholesterol levels. Because we eat too much meat, we are getting too much of these unhealthy fats.

What You Can Do

By limiting the amount of red meat that you eat, you can help to reduce the overall fat content in your diet.

You do need to get around about 35% of your calories from fat in order to remain healthy, but most of us exceed this figure on a daily basis.

You should make sure that you limit the portion sizes of meat eaten and that red meat is limited to no more than 2-3 meals a week.

Always choose leaner cuts and trim all visible fat from your meat before cooking it.

Action Plan

- Have at least one meatless dinner a week.

- Research alternative lean protein sources. Turkey and ostrich meat are both good options.

- When cooking fatty cuts of meat, use a griddle pan or grilling tray so the fat can drip off the meat.

Healthy Eating Habit 24: Stick to Similar Foods Daily

Most of us tend to be pretty erratic when it comes to what we eat.

We eat what we feel like eating. After all, variety is the spice of life, isn't it?

Research has actually found that eating similar foods every day is better for you.

What they have found is that people who limit their food choices to around about 4-5 different meal plans are naturally slimmer.

This is good for you for three basic reasons. First, you know what you will eat and know the calorie intake every day in advance, making calorie counting effortless. Second, you become more in tune with your body's needs throughout the day. And finally, our bodies like routines and habits.

What You Can Do

The idea here is not to eat the same boring food day in and day out.

You need to choose food that you enjoy from a limited range of menus.

Action Plan

- Find four or five recipes for breakfast that are healthy and balanced and that you really enjoy eating that all have the same basic calorie count.

- Do the same for lunch, dinner, and snacks.

- Now set up an eating plan with breakfast, lunch, dinner, and snacks, and interchange the basic meals however you want to.

Healthy Eating Habit 25: Cut Out Trans Fats

Trans-fats are one of the current villains in the food world and for very good reasons.

These are fats that have undergone a chemical transformation due to high heat or hydrogenation. As a result, they have become a lot more prone to oxidation and the production of free radicals.

Trans-fats are widely consumed and found just about everywhere.

Basically, any fat that is cannot handle high heat cooking can become a trans-fat. These include fats used extensively in the fast food industry such as sunflower and palm kernel oils.

What You Can Do

When cooking, use fats that are more stable under high heat conditions, such as coconut and olive oil.

Avoid any foods deep-fried in fat and any hydrogenated products. Most margarine and seed oils fall into this category.

Action Plan

- Switch from margarine back to butter.

- Cook with olive oil or coconut oil only.

- Find alternatives to deep fat frying.

- Avoid fast foods and only indulge occasionally.

Healthy Eating Habit 26: Keep Sodium Down & Potassium Up

Another common additive to foods is common table salt. It helps to act as a bit of a preservative and adds much needed flavor to processed foods.

As a result, you could be getting too much salt, even if you don't add it at the table or cook with it.

In fact, most of us eat too much salt every day.

Salt is necessary, but certainly not in the quantities that we use it. In fact, excessive salt intake can be very damaging to the hydrostatic balance in our bodies and can cause us to develop high blood pressure. It also puts extra pressure on the kidneys.

What You Can Do

Potassium can help to restore the balance lower blood pressure.

You need to decrease the amount of sodium consumed to less than 2,300 mg a day. At the same time, you need to increase the amount of potassium you consume.

Action Plan

- Do not add salt when cooking your food. If you must have salt, add it at the table. As with sugar, the taste for salty foods is one that is learned, and one that can be unlearned.

- Watch out for added salt in the foods you buy. Processed and canned foods tend to have a very high sodium content.

- Increase the amount of potassium you get in your diet. Bananas, citrus fruits, and yogurts are great sources of potassium.

Healthy Eating Habit 27: Spice Up Your Meals

There are fantastic benefits to eating more spices. Curry powder's main ingredient is turmeric. The anti-inflammatory properties of turmeric are 50% stronger than those of Vitamin-C. Cinnamon prevents your blood sugar from spiking and dipping, which can help you avoid cravings. And people who eat ginger on a daily basis experience 25% less exercise-induced muscle pain.

Other incredibly healthy spices include oregano, rosemary, nutmeg, cayenne, and cumin.

What You Can Do

Find ways to incorporate spices into every meal. Keep your spice rack full, and up to date. As you begin using more and more spices, you'll learn that they can be a fantastic substitute for sugar and salt.

Action Plan

- Invest in some good spices. Be sure to label them with the date you bought them so you know when to swap them out for new spices.

- Sprinkle cinnamon or nutmeg into your coffee in the morning instead of sugar.

- Cook chicken in a rub or oregano, rosemary, and a pinch of cayenne. You'll have a delicious, flavorful dinner with a lowered risk or ingesting cancer-causing amines that are produced when meat is cooked at high temperatures

- Choose to make curried rice instead of plain white rice.

Healthy Eating Habit 28: Keep Healthy Frozen Meals on Hand

As much as you'd like to plan every meal, it's just not practical. At 5:00 p.m. when you're starting to cook dinner, you might realize that you forgot an ingredient. You might remember that you have to be somewhere in one hour. You might even think, "I can't eat another bite of chicken," even though chicken is on the menu.

When these moments happen, don't panic or be forced to order a pizza. Have a back-up plan for the times when life interrupts your plans.

What You Can Do

Keep frozen meals in your freezer at all times. They can be meals you purchase from the store that aren't perfectly healthy, but are better than ordering take-out. Or you can make a big batch of a healthy soup or main dish that you keep for emergencies throughout the week.

Action Plan

- Fill your freezer with frozen vegetables, single serve meals, and one big entrée broken into single-portion containers.

- Keep an accurate count of what you have on hand. If you eat the freezer meal on Monday, don't wait a week to replace it.

Healthy Eating Habit 29: Work with A Friend

Everything is easier when you do it with a friend. Having someone else involved in your healthy-eating plans will help hold you accountable. People who have someone to report back to are more likely to stick to their goals because they know they will have to explain to someone why they failed. This is why weight loss programs with coaches are so popular. Having another person who has experienced, or is experiencing, the same thing can keep you both motivated and on track.

What You Can Do

Talk to a friend who is also on a diet or trying to stick to a healthy eating plan. Ask if they'd like to be your "diet partner." Odds are, they will be happy to have someone to work with.

Action Plan

- Set up a weekly meeting time when you will sit down with your friend and talk about your progress over the previous week.

- Share your food journals to keep each other accountable.

- Have an agreement that you can both call each other when you are tempted to make poor meal choices. Having someone to call to talk you out of pizza might be exactly what you need in order to make a better choice. Just the thoughts of having to make the call might be enough to dissuade you.

- Plan out designated "treat days," when you will go out and do something fun as a reward for your progress. This could be a food treat (Sunday breakfast once a month), but it doesn't have to be. It can be seeing a movie, going to an event that you both want to attend, or having a spa day. Just make sure it is something you both really want to do. This is your reward, after all.

Healthy Eating Habit 30: No Eating After 7 p.m.

Eating late into the night can lead to binging on unhealthy foods. Also, if you are still digesting food while you are trying to sleep, you will have lower quality sleep. Getting enough sleep at night is important for all of your bodily functions. Another benefit to eating earlier is that when you wake up, you will be hungry for breakfast. As mentioned before, it's very important to eat a good breakfast every day. This practice will help you do just that.

What You Can Do

Make an effort to not eat after 7:00 p.m. If you re going out with friends, or you have people over and eat late once in a while, it's not a huge problem. But as a rule, try to eat earlier in the day.

Action Plan

- Plan to have dinner at 5:30 p.m. or 6:00 p.m. Stop eating after dinner. If you want, have some tea or hot water with lemon.

Healthy Eating Habit 31: Eat Healthy Fats Every Day

You have probably been taught to avoid fats. But healthy fats are important to eat to maintain a healthy weight and for your body to be as healthy as it can be. The benefits to eating healthy fats are staggering. Eating healthy fats leads to better brain function, improved mood, less risk of depression and certain cancers, faster metabolism, a stronger immune system, improved skin and eye health, and easier weight loss. But not all fats are created equal. You already know you need Omega-3 fatty acids. You should get some healthy fats in every meal.

What You Can Do

Find ways to incorporate healthy fats into every meal. You don't need to eat a lot of healthy fats. Just a tablespoon of olive oil or a half an avocado here and there is sufficient. You already know you should be eating fish or taking an Omega-3 supplement. Add to this routine to incorporate fats in every meal.

Action Plan

- Cook vegetables in healthy oils like olive or coconut oil. Some vegetables are oil-soluble and some are water-soluble. If you don't cook the oil soluble vegetables in oil, you will not reap all of their benefits.

- Eat an avocado every day or every other day. You can cut it up to put on a salad, blend it into a smoothie, or stuff half of it with tuna salad.

Healthy Eating Habit 32: Incorporate Antioxidants into Your Diet

Antioxidants combat the free radicals that naturally form in the body. Antioxidants have been widely credited for warding off cancer, Alzheimer's disease, and heart disease. Our body naturally produces some antioxidants, but they are far outnumbered by free radicals. To maintain the balance, it's necessary to get antioxidants from outside sources as well. They are most commonly found in berries and vegetables.

What You Can Do

Find ways to incorporate antioxidants into your meals throughout the day. Berries and nuts are good sources of antioxidants, as are nuts, oranges, and beans.

Action Plan

- Add blueberries, blackberries, or raspberries to your oatmeal or cereal.

- Snack on a handful of pecans in the middle of the day.

- Drink a cup of green tea in the morning.

- Drink a glass of cherry juice before bed. Bonus: the melatonin in cherries will help you get a better night's sleep.

Healthy Eating Habit 33: Eat A Fiber-Rich Breakfast

Fiber is very important to dieters because it keeps you full. When you're full, you're less likely to snack on high calorie foods with low nutritional value. Adults should get between 25-35 grams of fiber each day, but most of us only get about 15.

What You Can Do

Start your day with a healthy dose of fiber. You should try to include it throughout the day, but breakfast is an easy place to start. Foods like leafy greens, beans, and whole grain all offer a few grams of fiber.

Action Plan

- Toss some spinach into your scrambled eggs to get more fiber.

- Eat a hearty serving of oatmeal for breakfast.

- If you're a fan of breakfast burritos, have one at least once a week for breakfast. Use black beans, veggies, and a whole-wheat tortilla to get a big dose of fiber.

Healthy Eating Habit 34: Switch to Whole Grains

Eating a diet rich in whole grains can reduce your risk of stroke, Type II Diabetes, heart disease, asthma, and a plethora of other diseases. And the wonderful thing is that whole grains are readily available in every grocery store.

What You Can Do

Spend some time analyzing the wheat sources that you eat on a daily basis. Would it be easy to switch any of them to a whole grain variety? Spend some time at your grocery store to find some healthy, delicious options.

Action Plan

- Eat whole grain cereals for breakfast.

- Switch to brown rice, instead of white rice.

- Eat whole grain bread if you are making a sandwich.

Healthy Eating Habit 35: Eat Fresh Foods

There is nothing healthier than whole, fresh foods. Fruits and vegetables lose some of their nutrients when they are cooked. The same is true of grains, nuts, and seeds.

What You Can Do

Eat as many fresh foods as possible. Try to eat unrefined grains and raw nuts and seeds.

Action Plan

- Incorporate lots of fruits and vegetables into your diet.

- Shop at farmer's markets when fresh produce is in season.

Healthy Eating Habit 36: Drink More Green Smoothies

One of the most important parts of a healthy diet is to get enough fruits and vegetables in your diet. But finding ways to incorporate nine servings each day can be difficult. One way to make this easier is to drink green smoothies. There are hundreds of varieties of green smoothies, but they all have one thing in common-they're packed with veggies. You can get 4-5 servings of vegetables in with just one smoothie!

What You Can Do

Find a way to start working green smoothies into your diet. They make an excellent breakfast because they provide a huge burst of energy from all the fresh veggies. They're also excellent mid-day snacks.

Action Plan

- Look up a few recipes to find some that sound good to you.

- Have a smoothie for breakfast at least once each week.

- Over time, start having smoothies once in a while for lunch or a snack.

- Try adding lemon or berries to your smoothies for a little sweetness.

A Special Gift Just For YOU

FOR A LIMITED TIME ONLY – Get Linda's best-selling book *"Quick & Easy Weight Loss: 97 Scientifically Proven Tips Even For Those With Busy Schedules!"* absolutely FREE!

Readers who have read this bonus book along with this book have seen the greatest changes in their weight loss both *FAST & EASILY* and have improved overall fitness levels – so it is *highly recommended* to get this bonus book.

Once again, as a big thank-you for downloading this book, I'd like to offer it to you *100% FREE for a LIMITED TIME ONLY!*

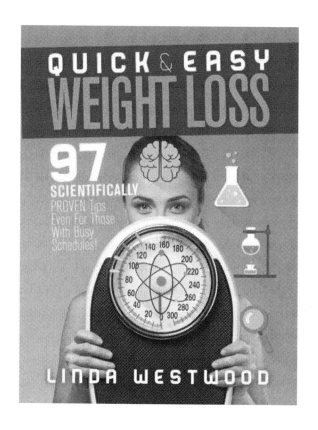

Get your free copy at:

TopFitnessAdvice.com/Bonus

Healthy Eating Habit 37: Don't Give Anything Up

What if someone told you that you were never allowed to eat another brownie. For the rest of your life, you were forbidden from eating them. What would you say? Probably, you'd immediately want a brownie. And if not, you'd really want one later. Taking certain foods off the menu indefinitely is not only impractical, but it's not necessary. It's okay to indulge every once in a while. In fact, it's essential in order to stay on track in the long run. So, don't give anything up!

What You Can Do

Know what your "indulgence foods," are. These are the foods that you absolutely LOVE, but you know you shouldn't eat very often. Maybe you could never part with pizza or ice cream. Maybe it's steak or cheese. Whatever it is, learn what a single portion is. Make it very clear to yourself that you are allowed to eat those foods, but you are choosing not to eat them very often.

Action Plan

- Have a designated day or meal when you eat these "indulgence foods."

- Be sure to only eat one normally sized portions.

Healthy Eating Habit 38: Don't Count Calories

Counting calories is nowhere near as effective in practice as it is in theory. Sure, eating fewer calories will cause you to lose weight, but the best way to stay trim or lose weight is to cut fat, increase your protein intake, and switch to healthy, unrefined carbs.

When you just focus on counting calories, you miss out on a huge piece of your healthy eating plan. You fail to take into account, which foods are good for you and which are horrible empty calories. An apple and a low carb beer both have about 100 calories. Is one equal to the other? Certainly, not.

What You Can Do

Skip the urge to count calories. A healthy diet of whole grains, fruits and vegetables, and low fat proteins can actually lead to a high caloric intake. This isn't necessarily a bad thing.

Action Plan

- If you must count calories, also records which calories came from fat, carbs, protein, etc. This will give you a more accurate picture of what you are consuming.

- Try to focus on eating healthy, whole foods instead or worrying about the calorie count.

Healthy Eating Habit 39: Have A Prep-Day

You already know you should do your grocery shopping once a week. But a prep day is about more than grocery shopping. It's about using that day to do all that you can to make the rest of the week easier.

What You Can Do

Set aside one day of the week to prepare for the week ahead. Use this day to do as much prep work as possible. This will make your week run more smoothly, and you will be better prepared for any last minute changes.

Action Plan

- Fill zip lock bags with single servings of snacks. Keep them in one place so you can easily find snacks when you need them.

- Make a big batch of a healthy soup. Divide it into portion-sized containers, and put them in the freezer for emergency meals when you aren't able to stick to your plan.

- Cut up all of the vegetables you will need later in the week.

Healthy Eating Habit 40: Get A Slow Cooker

There are very few things as satisfying as coming home to a fully prepared dinner. The house smells wonderful, and you know that all you have to do is get a plate or a bowl, and enjoy your home-cooked meal.

Slow cookers are especially helpful when you are trying to stick to a diet because they offer so much versatility. You can make stews, meats, vegetarian dishes, breakfast, lunch, and dinner. And because the food cooks slowly at a low temperature, you don't need to add many extras to make everything taste delicious. The flavors have enough time to really meld together.

What You Can Do

Plan to incorporate slow cooked meals into your meal plan at least once a week. You can make breakfast the night before, and wake up to a healthy slow cooked oatmeal, or you can prepare dinner for a night when you know you won't have the time or motivation to cook.

Action Plan

- Buy a slow cooker cookbook, or look up some recipes online. Choose 5 or 6 that look good to you, and incorporate them into your meal plan.

- Prep your ingredients the night before you will need them. You're more likely to stick to your meal plan if you don't have to chop veggies in the morning when you're running out the door.

Healthy Eating Habit 41: Use The 80/20 Rule

You may have heard of the 80/20 Rule as it relates to talking and listening. You are supposed to listen 80% of the time and talk 20% of the time. But there is also an application of the rule in regards to eating.

What You Can Do

There are two applications for the 80/20 rule. You can eat until you are 80% full, and allow yourself to remain 20% hungry each time you eat.

You can also eat healthy, nutritious foods 80% of the time, and allow yourself to splurge 20% of the time.

Action Plan

- Allow yourself one splurge day each week. Alternatively, you can just keep in mind that the occasional splurge is ok. Just don't splurge every day.

- Stop eating while you are still a little bit hungry. Your food will continue to process, making you feel full later. If you eat until you feel full, you will actually have overeaten.

Healthy Eating Habit 42: Drink Water in The Morning

You already know the important of getting enough water in your diet. Literally every one of your organs relies on water to function. But trying to work in the right amount can be difficult.

One of the best ways to drink enough water is to drink it in the morning before you leave your house. Once the day gets going, it can be hard to remember to drink. So, make it easy on yourself by getting a solid start in the morning.

What You Can Do

Find ways to incorporate water into your morning routine. Aim to get 16-24 ounces in before you leave the house. You can also keep a bottle of water in the car or your purse for your morning commute.

Action Plan

- Set out a large glass of water next to your bed. First thing in the morning, drink the glass of water.

- Set out another large glass of water next to the sink. In the morning, when you wake up to brush your teeth, drink two full glasses.

- Now you've gotten three glasses of water in your body before even leaving the house!

Healthy Eating Habit 43: Record How You Feel After Each Meal

This isn't the same as keeping a food diary. While a food diary keeps track of what you eat so you are more accountable, a record of your how you feel before and after each meal will help you identify which foods give you energy, and which foods leave you hungry an hour later.

What You Can Do

Keep a running record of how you feel before every meal. Rate your hunger level, emotions, and cravings. Once you have had a meal, rate your hunger level again.

Also, write down how you feel. Are you satisfied? Are you sluggish? If anything strange happens later (indigestion, anger, upset stomach), write it down. Over time, you'll be able to have a better idea of how your body reacts to different foods.

Action Plan

- Buy a second diary to track your emotions, or use a food tracker app.

- Rate your hunger on a scale of 1-10 before and after each meal and snack.

- Keep a running list of any foods that make you particularly energized and any that leave you in a slump.

- Keep track of how you feel after drinking water, caffeinated beverages, and alcohol, and how you feel after eating sugary or salty foods.

Healthy Eating Habit 44: Cut Back on Alcohol

There are many studies that show that one glass of red wine every day improves overall health and may prevent heart disease. However, drinking in excess is damaging to every part of your body.

Drinking causes liver disease, dehydration, and weight gain (among a very long list of other negative effects). If you are trying to go on a "diet," or just eat healthier on a daily basis, it's important to cut out or limit the consumption of alcohol.

What You Can Do

Aim to cut back your drinking to no more than one alcoholic beverage per day (if you are drinking it for the health benefits). If you are drinking hard alcohol or beer, aim to cut it out completely, or have a drink as an occasional indulgence.

Action Plan

- Learn what one portion of alcohol is. One serving of hard alcohol is one ounce. One 12 oz. beer or one 4-6 oz. glass of wine are also single servings.

- If you are going out with friends, have a wine spritzer or a vodka soda (with just one shot of vodka). They are both low calorie drinks. You can also have a cranberry juice with soda water and a lime wedge. It's fancy and delicious, and you won't feel like you have to miss out on a night with your friends.

Healthy Eating Habit 45: Shop the Perimeter of The Store

Al the best things in the grocery store are on the outside edges. The fresh fruits and vegetables, bulk foods, and whole grains are all along the perimeter. All of the processed and junk food is in the middle of the store.

What You Can Do

Do your best to shop along the outside of the store. Limit your "middle" purchases to just a few items (if any).

Action Plan

- When making your grocery list, imagine your grocery store. When you're tempted to add processed items, think twice about whether or not you need those.

- If you really want something form the middle of the store, try to think of a way you can make that same item using "perimeter" foods.

Healthy Eating Habit 46: Learn A Go-To Recipe

Remember your mom's apple pie or your grandma's pot roast? They didn't need a recipe because they had made it a thousand times. It was their signature dish. The benefits of having a "signature dish" are tremendous.

You can save time by not having to plan out the recipe, you can keep the ingredients in your house all the time in case you need a fast meal, and you can share it with your friends and family as your special meal. When you're trying to eat healthy, having a go-to signature meal is even more important.

You can make a fast healthy meal on nights when you forget to meal plan. You can also have a healthy choice to bring to parties.

What You Can Do

Come up with several go-to recipes that you can make quickly and easily. Ideally, they should be only a few ingredients, and you should be able to make them in a pinch.

Action Plan

- Go online to find a fast recipe that you love.

- Make the recipe a few times until you are very comfortable with it and you don't have to follow the directions anymore.

- Find another recipe that you can share at parties. This should be a salad, a healthy casserole, or a hearty soup.

Healthy Eating Habit 47: Plan for The Holidays

The holidays can present a real dilemma for people trying to stick to a healthy diet. It seems like you're constantly surrounded by chocolate, meat, cheese, alcohol, and candy. You certainly don't want to overindulge in all that heavy food. But you also don't want to have to skip every party you're invited to.

What You Can Do

Have a plan before you go to the party. Have a healthy dinner before you arrive so you're not hungry. You'll be less tempted when you're full. You can also offer to bring a dish that everyone will love.

Action Plan

- Allow yourself one treat at each party. It might be eggnog with brandy or some pumpkin pie - but limit it to just one slice.

- Call the host ahead of time to thank him for the invitation. Let him know you're on a special diet, and you'd love to bring a dish to share with everyone. Ask what would go well with their selection.

Healthy Eating Habit 48: Eat Your Leafy Greens

Leafy greens are rich in vitamin K, which helps your blood clot. It also helps your body prevent the effects that aging has on your cells. One serving of raw leafy greens gives you your daily does of vitamin k.

One cup of kale gives you six times your daily requirement! Leafy greens are also rich in calcium. If you're trying to cut back on dairy, but you don't want to miss out on the calcium it provides, kick up your intake of leafy green vegetables.

What You Can Do

Aim to get at least 3 servings of leafy green vegetables each day. If you eat them raw, one cup constitutes a serving. If you cook them, you only need a half-cup per serving.

Action Plan

- Identify a few leafy green vegetables that you either really like, or are willing to deal with.

- Blend leafy greens into a smoothie in the morning.

- Add some spinach to your scrambled eggs.

Healthy Eating Habit 49: Get Some Sunshine

Vitamin D is essential to your body because it aids in the absorption of calcium. If you don't have adequate Vitamin D in your diet, your body will not be able to process calcium. That's why so many products, like cereal, soymilk, and orange juice, are Vitamin-D fortified.

In addition to helping absorb calcium, Vitamin-D also helps maintain teeth and bone strength and is partially credited with fending off cancer and multiple sclerosis. Unfortunately, it's very difficult to get enough Vitamin-D from foods alone. You can take a supplement. But the best way to get your daily dose of Vitamin-D is to expose your bare skin to the sun.

What You Can Do

Aim to get 20-25 minutes of sun exposure each day. You can't get it through a window.

Action Plan

- Sip your morning coffee in the sunlight outside.

- Get out of the office for a 15-minute walk in the middle of the day.

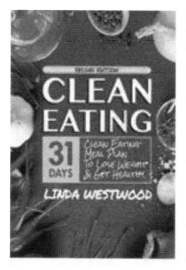
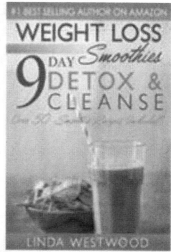
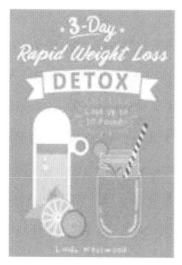
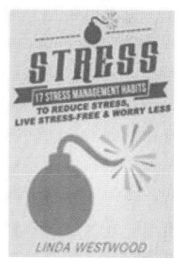

Check out Linda's best selling books at:

TopFitnessAdvice.com/go/books

Healthy Eating Habit 50: Eat Dessert First

Some might argue that the best part of any meal is dessert. Those people are not wrong. However, you certainly don't want to eat dessert every night. Dessert should be an indulgence that you allow yourself every once in a while.

What You Can Do

On nights when you do allow yourself dessert, if can be tempting to over-indulge. After all, you don't get to eat dessert every day; you might as well go big or go home! Unfortunately, if you do that, you will see that your healthy eating efforts have been in vain.

Instead, limit yourself to one small serving of dessert, and eat it *before* you eat your meal. This will do a few things. One, it will make it feel like an even bigger treat.

Second, it will make you less likely to over indulge. There's no need to eat two pieces of cake before you start your dinner. And eating a second piece of cake after dinner when you already had one before dinner? You can fight that craving.

Action Plan

- Eat only one serving of your dessert before you eat your dinner.

- Do not make a whole cake or pie. Try to buy just one piece from a bakery so you won't be tempted with the leftovers.

Healthy Eating Habit 51: Pack A Lunch

If you work in an office, lunchtime can be the hardest part of your day to plan. You can easily get a healthy breakfast at home, and you can meal plan so you always know what's going to be on the menu for dinner, but lunch offers so many opportunities to give into temptation.

A co-worker could bring donuts to the office. You might work near a restaurant, or you might have to walk past a vending machine every day. When it's the middle of the day, and you're hungry, it can be very hard to make healthy choices. Be prepared by packing a lunch.

What You Can Do

Bring a lunch to work every day, with no exceptions. Avoid the vending machine by leaving your change purse at home. And do all you can to ignore the donuts or other snacks in the break room.

Action Plan

- Invest in a good lunchbox. You can get a sturdy one to divide your lunch into different compartments.

- Make your lunch the night before you go to work, and leave yourself a note on the front door so you don't forget to bring it.

- Keep healthy snacks in your desk drawer for days when you're still hungry after eating your lunch.

Healthy Eating Habit 52: Go for A Walk

Walking is good for you for so many reasons. Just getting 10,000 steps each day is an easy way to maintain a healthy weight. Walking aids in digestion, and prevents or relieves stress. It clears your mind and offers a full body workout. A regular walking routine should be a part of any healthy eating plan.

What You Can Do

Aim to get 10,000 steps in every day. To do this, you can either buy a pedometer or download an app that tracks your steps.

Action Plan

- Take a 30-45-minute walk every evening after dinner.

- Take a walk first thing in the morning to get a little exercise and kick-start your day.

Healthy Eating Habit 53: Chew Gum

There are some surprising health benefits associated with chewing gum. Each person is different and will have a different result from chewing gum. But overall, chewing gum has been shown to improve memory, reduce stress, increase concentration and focus, lose weight, and improve oral health.

With so many wonderful benefits, it makes sense to chew gum. Just make sure to choose the sugar free variety so you're not adding unnecessary sugar to your diet.

What You Can Do

Keep a pack of gum in your purse, car, or desk drawer. Chew it while you're studying or working on important projects to improve focus and alertness.

Action Plan

- If you're bored, reach for a stick of gum instead of a snack. Of course, if you're hungry, reach for a snack.

- Chew gum after meals to make your mouth feel clean, and to help fight off cravings. Studies have shown that people are less likely to snack when their mouths feel clean, like right after brushing your teeth or chewing gum.

Healthy Eating Habit 54: Find Substitutes for Your Favorite Indulgences

We all have cravings. At midnight, you must have pizza! At 3:00 p.m., you hit a slump and reach for the chocolate. Your cravings aren't likely to go away anytime soon. Over time, you can train your body to crave healthy foods, but until that day comes, you need a better plan of action than giving in every time.

What You Can Do

Figure out what it is that you crave. Do you love sugar? Do you prefer salty or savory snacks? Do you need to hear that crunch when you chew? Identify what you crave the most, and find healthy ways to work it into your diet.

Action Plan

- Substitute kale chips for potato chips.

- Bake apples in the oven on low heat, and sprinkle them with cinnamon to fight off a sugar craving.

- Eat some Greek yogurt with blueberries instead of ice cream.

Healthy Eating Habit 55: Get Enough Sleep

Sleep is the cornerstone of a healthy life. People who get enough sleep are proven to be healthier, thinner, and happier. Most people need 8 hours of sleep. You might need 7 or 9.

Lack of sleep causes aggravation, which might lead to poor eating habits. You will also likely be tired, which could cause you to reach for a sugary, high calorie snack like a candy bar. This will give you a quick burst of energy, but it will leave you feeling even worse later.

What You Can Do

Make it a point to get enough sleep every night. Turn off all technology devices 30 minutes before bed to help you get into the right mood to fall asleep. Read a book or do another relaxing activity to quiet your mind. Block out as much light as possible from your bedroom. You will sleep best in a very dark room.

Action Plan

- Go to bed at a reasonable hour. Determine what time you need to be awake, and make sure you are in bed at least 8 hours before that time. It might take some time to get used to this schedule, but eventually you will go to sleep with ease.

- Get a better alarm clock. Some smart phone apps are designed to wake you up when you are most easily awakened. These apps can help you wake more readily and with more energy.

- Don't consumer alcohol, caffeine, or sugary foods within a few hours of bedtime. These things will make it harder to fall asleep, and you will likely have lower-quality sleep than when you avoid these items.

Healthy Eating Habit 56: Learn to Love Soup

When the weather is cold and it's dark outside, nothing hits the spot quite like a hot bowl of soup. Maybe you're a tomato soup with grilled cheese kind of person. Or maybe you have a favorite childhood recipe.

It's easy to see the appeal of soup on a cold winter's night. But what about the rest of the time? Soup is an excellent meal for any time of year. Even in the heat of summer, you can make cold cucumber soup, gazpacho, or even a standard hot soup.

Soup is low-calorie, easy to make, and freezer friendly. If you're trying to eat a healthy diet, soup is a much have staple.

What You Can Do

Find ways to incorporate soup into your diet on a regular basis. You can make it for a freezer swap or for yourself. Load your soup up with veggies, and use spices instead of salt to enhance the flavor.

Action Plan

- Look up 4-5 soup recipes that you'd like to try. They can be new recipes or old favorites.

- Add at least two of these to your meal plan each week. Soup can be an easy lunch, a slow cooked stew, or a quick meal in the evening.

- Be sure to make your own soup. Canned soups are full of sodium and sugar.

- Make a big batch of soup on your prep day. Divide it into individual containers, and put them in the freezer for emergency meals.

Healthy Eating Habit 57: Take Your Vitamins

It's important to get your daily requirement of vitamins and minerals. Vitamins keep your body healthy and help to improve muscle and body functions.

What You Can Do

Talk to your doctor to learn if there are any vitamins you should be taking beyond a once a day multi-vitamin. Depending on your personal health, you may need a boost of specific vitamins.

Action Plan

- Take a once-a-day multi-vitamin in the morning with a big glass of water.

- Pay attention to any symptoms that may be indicative of needing a vitamin supplement. For instance, if you are a vegan, you should be taking a B12 every day.

Last Chance to Get YOUR Bonus!

FOR A LIMITED TIME ONLY – Get Linda's best-selling book *"Quick & Easy Weight Loss: 97 Scientifically Proven Tips Even For Those With Busy Schedules!"* absolutely FREE!

Readers who have read this bonus book along with this book have seen the greatest changes in their weight loss both *FAST & EASILY* and have improved overall fitness levels – so it is *highly recommended* to get this bonus book.

Once again, as a big thank-you for downloading this book, I'd like to offer it to you *100% FREE for a LIMITED TIME ONLY!*

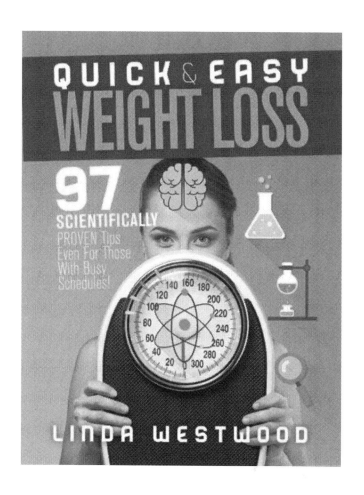

To download your FREE book, go to:

TopFitnessAdvice.com/Bonus

Healthy Eating Habit 58: Have A Freezer Swap

A freezer swap is an event where two or more people get together with individually portioned frozen meals (preferably home cooked).

Then, everybody swaps meals! It's a great way to get your friends involved in a healthy eating plan. It will also save you money because you only have to buy ingredients for one meal, and make a big batch (rather than buying ingredients for several meals and making smaller portions).

What You Can Do

Arrange a freezer swap of your own. Invite friends to join whom either have the same dietary preferences as you or who are willing to work around your requirements. Schedule the swap once a week.

Action Plan

- Select a group of friends who are willing to participate on a weekly or semi-weekly basis.

- Assign each person a meal. Everyone can bring an entree, or you can have some people bring breakfast, some bring lunch, and some bring dinner.

- Each person should make a big batch of their chosen entrée and divide it into enough servings so that each person in the swap can take home one or two.

- Once you get to the swap, divide up the meals.

- Plan to meet twice or four times per month.

- Be sure to factor the freezer swap into your weekly grocery list.

Healthy Eating Habit 59: Buy Smaller Dishes

It's likely that as a child, you were told to "clear your plate." Psychologically, we are still wired to do that. We will put more food on our plates when we have bigger plates to fill, and we will consume more food because we still feel the need to eat everything on the plate.

Buying smaller plates can help u eat less by tricking the body into thinking it's getting more food than it is actually getting.

What You Can Do

Get some smaller plates so you can still fill them, but you won't end up overeating.

Action Plan

- Go to the store, and buy some smaller plates.

- Only fill your plate one time.

- You can do the same thing with dessert plates and wine glasses. The smaller the dishes are, the less likely you will be to over indulge.

Final Words

I would like to thank you for downloading my book and I hope I have been able to help you and educate you about something new.

If you have enjoyed this book and would like to share your positive thoughts, could you please take 30 seconds of your time to go back and give me a review on my Amazon book page!

I greatly appreciate seeing these reviews because it helps me share my hard work!

Again, thank you and I wish you all the best with your weight loss journey!

Disclaimer

This book and related sites provide wellness management information in an informative and educational manner only, with information that is general in nature and that is not specific to you, the reader. The contents of this site are intended to assist you and other readers in your personal wellness efforts. Consult your physician regarding the applicability of any information provided in our sites to you.

Nothing in this book should be construed as personal advices or diagnosis, and must not be used in this manner. The information provided about conditions is general in nature. This information does not cover all possible uses, actions, precautions, side effects, or interactions of medicines, or medical procedures. The information in this site should not be considered as complete and does not cover all diseases, ailments, physical conditions, or their treatment.

You should **consult with your physician before beginning any exercise, weight loss, or healthcare program**. This book **should not** be used in place of a call or visit to a competent health-care professional. You should consult a health care professional before adopting any of the suggestions in this book or before drawing inferences from it.

Any decision regarding treatment and medication for your condition should be made with the advice and consultation of a qualified health care professional. If you have, or suspect you have, a health-care problem, then you should immediately contact a qualified health care professional for treatment.

No Warranties: The authors and publishers don't guarantee or warrant the quality, accuracy, completeness, timeliness, appropriateness or suitability of the information in this book, or of any product or services referenced by this site.

The information in this site is provided on an "as is" basis and the authors and publishers make no representations or warranties of any kind with respect to this information. This site may contain inaccuracies, typographical errors, or other errors.

Liability Disclaimer: The publishers, authors, and other parties involved in the creation, production, provision of information, or delivery of this site specifically disclaim any responsibility, and shall not be held liable for any damages, claims, injuries, losses, liabilities, costs, or obligations including any direct, indirect, special, incidental, or consequences damages (collectively known as "Damages") whatsoever and howsoever caused, arising out of, or in connection with the use or misuse of the site and the information contained within it, whether such Damages arise in contract, tort, negligence, equity, statute law, or by way of other legal theory.

18527324R00064

Printed in Great Britain
by Amazon